DIABETES COOKBOOK AND MEAL PLAN

Managing Blood Sugar through Smart Nutrition

A Comprehensive Guide To Supporting Diabetic Patients With Breakfast Options, Lunch Ideas, Dinner Recipes, Healthy Snack Choices, Beverage Recommendations, Special Occasion Menus, And Good Eating Ideas For The Newly Diagnosed

Dr. Marley Marian

Table of Contents

Chapter One

Introduction

Diabetes is a chronic disorder that causes high blood sugar levels owing to the body's inability to effectively use or make insulin. It affects millions of people throughout the globe and must be managed carefully to avoid consequences. Diabetes management relies heavily on nutrition since dietary choices have a direct influence on blood sugar levels.

Understanding diabetes

Diabetes is classified into many types, the most common of which are Type 1 and Type 2. Type 1 diabetes is an autoimmune disease in which the body destroys its insulin-producing cells, necessitating lifelong insulin injections. Type 2 diabetes is primarily caused by insulin resistance, which occurs when the body's cells become resistant to insulin or produce insufficient insulin. Diet, activity, and weight are all important risk factors for Type 2 diabetes.

The significance of nutrition in managing diabetes

1. Controlling Blood Sugar Levels: Carbohydrates have a substantial influence on blood sugar levels. Choosing complex carbs high in fiber, such as whole grains, fruits, and vegetables, may help regulate blood sugar levels.

2. Managing Weight: Maintaining a healthy weight is critical for diabetes management. A nutrient-dense diet and portion management aid in achieving and maintaining a healthy weight.

3. Preventing Complications: A good diet reduces the risk of diabetes-related complications such as heart disease, nerve damage, and kidney failure.

4. Improving Insulin Sensitivity: Certain meals, such as leafy greens, nuts, and fatty fish, may help cells absorb glucose from the circulation.

5. Promoting Heart Health: Diabetes raises the risk of heart disease. A diet low in saturated fats, cholesterol,

and salt, but rich in fiber, lean proteins, and healthy fats, promotes cardiovascular health.

6. Increasing Energy Levels: Balanced meals give consistent energy throughout the day, avoiding energy dumps and excessive hunger, which may lead to bad eating choices.

7. Supporting Overall Health: A proper diet promotes the immune system, bone health, and mental well-being, all of which are critical components of diabetes control.

8. Improving Blood Pressure regulation: A diet rich in fruits, vegetables, and whole grains that is low in salt helps regulate blood pressure, lowering the risk of problems associated with high blood pressure in diabetes.

9. Improving Lipid Profile: Healthy fats, such as omega-3 fatty acids found in fish, nuts, and seeds, may help to reduce triglyceride levels and increase HDL (good) cholesterol.

10. Providing Structure and Routine: Having regular meal times and consistent carbohydrate consumption

helps to normalize blood sugar levels and improves diabetes control.

Getting started with smart nutrition

Smart nutrition for diabetes control is following a well-balanced diet that emphasizes whole foods and mindful eating. Here are some suggestions to get started:

1. meal Control: Keep track of your meal amounts to avoid overeating and properly regulate blood sugar levels.

2. Macronutrient Balancing: Aim for a carbohydrate, protein, and fat balance in each meal to offer long-lasting energy and avoid blood sugar spikes.

3. Choosing Whole Foods: Opt for whole, unprocessed foods like fruits, vegetables, lean meats, whole grains, and healthy fats over processed and refined meals.

4. Monitoring Carbohydrate Intake: Keep track of the kind and quantity of carbohydrates you ingest, concentrating on complex carbs with high fiber content and reducing simple sugars.

5. Staying Hydrated: Drink enough of water throughout the day to keep your body hydrated and functioning properly.

Ingredients to Cook for Diabetes Patients

Diabetes is a disorder in which blood sugar levels must be carefully managed via diet, exercise, and, in some cases, medication. When preparing meals for diabetics, it's critical to choose products that won't raise blood sugar levels while yet delivering necessary nutrients. Here's a thorough list of diabetes-friendly substances, along with their functions:

1. Whole grains:

• Examples include quinoa, brown rice, oats, and barley.

• Whole grains include fiber, which slows glucose absorption and prevents blood sugar rises. They also provide critical elements such as vitamins, minerals, and antioxidants.

2. Lean proteins:

• Examples include skinless fowl, fish, tofu, legumes (beans and lentils), and lean cuts of beef or pig.

• Proteins decrease carbohydrate digestion and absorption, hence stabilizing blood sugar levels. They also increase satiety and improve muscular health.

3. Nonstarchy Vegetables:

• Examples include spinach, broccoli, peppers, cauliflower, and Brussels sprouts.

• Non-starchy veggies include large amounts of fiber, vitamins, and minerals while being low in carbs and calories. They aid in blood sugar regulation, support weight management, and lower the risk of chronic illnesses.

4. Healthy fats:

• Examples include avocado, almonds, seeds, olive oil, and fatty fish (e.g., salmon and mackerel).

• Healthy fats provide vital fatty acids and fat-soluble vitamins. They also increase insulin sensitivity, decrease inflammation, and promote cardiovascular health.

5. Low-Glycemic Fruit:

• Examples include strawberries, blueberries, raspberries, apples, and citrus fruits.

• Low-glycemic fruits absorb sugars more slowly, resulting in modest rises in blood sugar levels. They also deliver vitamins, minerals, and antioxidants without generating sudden glucose increases.

6. Herbs and spices:

• Examples include cinnamon, turmeric, garlic, ginger, and basil.

• Herbs and spices provide flavor to foods without using excessive salt, sugar, or harmful fats. Some spices, such as cinnamon, may even enhance insulin sensitivity and reduce blood sugar levels.

7. Low-fat dairy and dairy alternatives:

• Examples include Greek yogurt, unsweetened almond milk, and low-fat cheese.

• Low-fat dairy products include calcium, protein, and vitamin D without added saturated fats. They promote bone health and may help control blood pressure.

8. Sweeteners:

• Examples include Stevia, Erythritol, and Monk Fruit Extract.

• These alternative sweeteners deliver sweetness without raising blood sugar levels. They may be used in moderation to fulfill sweet desires while maintaining glycemic control.

9. Flax with Chia Seeds:

• The seeds are high in fiber, omega-3 fatty acids, and antioxidants. They aid in controlling blood sugar, boosting heart health, and promoting digestive regularity.

10. Vinegar:

• Vinegar, particularly apple cider vinegar, may enhance insulin sensitivity and reduce blood sugar levels after meals. It may be used in salad dressings and marinades.

11. Water:

• Staying hydrated is essential for diabetics to avoid dehydration, manage blood sugar levels, and promote kidney function. Water is the greatest option for hydration, however herbal teas and infused water may also be enjoyed.

Chapter Two

Breakfast Options For Diabetics

1. Plain oats sprinkled with berries and almonds make for a fiber-rich breakfast that helps to keep blood sugar levels stable.

2. Greek Yogurt Parfait: Combine Greek yogurt, berries, and granola for a protein-packed breakfast that will keep you satisfied.

3. Vegetable Omelette: Make an omelet with spinach, tomatoes, and bell peppers for a low-carb, high-protein meal.

4. Spread mashed avocado over whole grain bread for a nutrient-dense breakfast high in healthy fats and fiber.

5. Smoothie: For a quick and nutritious breakfast, combine leafy greens, berries, protein powder, and unsweetened almond milk.

1. Quinoa Salad: For a satisfying and healthy meal, mix quinoa with veggies, legumes, and a lean protein source such as grilled chicken or tofu.

2. Grilled Chicken Wrap: Wrap grilled chicken, lettuce, tomatoes, and hummus in a whole-grain tortilla for a nutritious and portable lunch.

3. Salmon Salad: For a heart-healthy meal, top mixed greens with grilled salmon, avocado, almonds, and vinaigrette dressing.

4. Vegetable Stir-Fry: Cook mixed veggies with tofu or shrimp and serve over brown rice for a filling and low-glycemic meal.

5. Turkey & Veggie Wrap: Wrap turkey slices, avocado, and mixed veggies in a whole wheat wrap for a light yet filling lunch option.

Dinner Recipes For Diabetic-Friendly Meals

1. Grilled Fish with Roasted Vegetables: Serve fish fillets with roasted vegetables seasoned with herbs and olive oil for a tasty and healthy supper.

2. Chicken and Vegetable Skewers: Thread chicken chunks and a variety of veggies onto skewers, grill or bake, and serve with quinoa or brown rice for a complete dinner.

3. Vegetable Curry: Simmer mixed veggies in a tasty curry sauce prepared with coconut milk and spices, then serve over cauliflower rice for a low-carb supper.

4. Stuffed Bell Peppers: Fill bell peppers with a combination of lean ground turkey, quinoa, veggies, and seasonings, bake until soft, and serve with a side salad for a filling supper.

5. Zucchini Noodles with Turkey Bolognese: For a lighter pasta night, spiralize zucchini and top with turkey

bolognese sauce prepared with lean ground turkey and marinara sauce. Garnish with grated Parmesan cheese.

Finally, treating diabetes via diet is critical for regulating blood sugar levels, avoiding complications, and improving general health and well-being. Individuals with diabetes may enhance their quality of life by making wise food choices and integrating balanced meals into their daily routines.

10 Healthy Snack Options To Manage Blood Sugar Levels

1. Greek Yogurt with Berries:

• Step 1: Gather items, including Greek yogurt and fresh berries.

• Step 2: In a dish, place one serving of Greek yogurt.

• Step 3: Wash and place fresh berries on top.

• Step 4: Enjoy the creamy smoothness and natural sweetness without raising blood sugar.

2. Vegetable Sticks with Hummus

• Step 1: Wash and chop fresh veggies into sticks, including carrots, cucumbers, and bell peppers.

• Step 2: Prepare or buy hummus.

• Step 3: Dip veggie sticks in hummus for a crisp and delicious snack.

3. Nut & Seed Mix:

• Step 1: Mix nuts and seeds, including almonds, walnuts, and pumpkin seeds.

• Step 2: Divide single portions into tiny containers for convenient grab-and-go.

• Step 3: Consume protein and healthy fats to balance blood sugar levels.

4. Avocado with Whole Grain Crackers:

• Step 1: Toast whole grain crackers.

• Step 2: Spread mashed avocado on top of crackers.

• Step 3: Add salt and pepper for taste.

• Step 4: Enjoy the creamy, fiber-rich snack.

5. Cottage Cheese and Pineapple:

• Step 1: Place cottage cheese in a bowl.

• Step 2: Include fresh pineapple pieces.

• Step 3: Combine ingredients for a protein-rich snack with a dash of sweetness.

6. Hardboiled Eggs:

• Step 1: Cook eggs until hard-cooked.

• Step 2: Peel and eat as a protein-rich snack.

• Step 3: Season with salt and pepper as required.

7. Edamame pods:

• Step 1: Cook or steam the edamame pods until soft.

• Step 2: Season with a pinch of sea salt.

• Step 3: Shell and pop the beans for a healthful, low-carb snack.

8. Apple Slices with Peanut Butter:

• Step 1: Cut an apple into wedges.

• Step 2: Add natural peanut butter to each slice.

• Step 3: Enjoy a pleasant snack with a sweet and nutty flavor.

9. Cherry tomatoes with mozzarella:

• Step 1: Wash cherry tomatoes and slice fresh mozzarella cheese.

• Step 2: Skewer a tomato and a chunk of mozzarella on toothpicks.

• Step 3: Add balsamic glaze if desired.

10. Cucumber Roll-ups:

• Begin by slicing cucumbers lengthwise into thin strips with a mandolin.

• Step 2: Spread cream cheese or hummus onto each strip.

• Step 3: Roll and fasten with a toothpick for a low-carb, refreshing snack.

10 Drink Recommendations for Diabetics:

1. Water and Lemon:

• Step 1: Add fresh lemon juice to a glass of water.

• Step 2: Stir and enjoy the delicious and hydrating drink.

2. Green Tea:

• Step 1: Steep the green tea bag in boiling water for 3-5 minutes.

• Step 2: Remove the tea bag and drink the antioxidant-rich brew.

3. Herbal tea infusions:

• Step 1: Select herbal teas, such as chamomile or peppermint.

• Step 2: Steep in boiling water for 5-7 min.

• Step 3: Strain and enjoy the relaxing benefits.

4. Sparkling water with a splash of lime

• Step 1: Add sparkling water to a glass.

• Step 2: Add fresh lime juice for a tangy taste.

• Step 3: Optionally add ice cubes for a refreshing effervescent drink.

5. Vegetable Juice Blend:

• Step 1: Juice low-glycemic veggies such as spinach, cucumber, and celery.

• Step 2: Pour into a glass and enjoy the nutrient-rich drink.

6. Iced Herbal Infusion:

• Step 1: Make herbal tea and chill it to room temperature.

• Step 2: To enhance taste, add ice cubes and a piece of lemon or cucumber.

• Step 3: Drink the cooling and hydrating drink.

7. Almond Milk Latte.

• Step 1: Steam almond milk until foamy.

• Step 2: Make a shot of espresso or strong coffee.

• Step 3: Add almond milk to the coffee for a creamy, caffeinated boost.

8. Coconut Water:

• Step 1: Open a fresh coconut or buy prepared coconut water.

• Pour into a glass with ice for a hydrating and electrolyte-rich drink.

9. Low-Sugar Smoothies

• Step 1: Combine spinach, berries, avocado, and unsweetened almond milk.

• Step 2: Add ice cubes to thicken and chill.

• Step 3: Enjoy a healthy and full smoothie without raising blood sugar levels.

10. Homemade infused water:

• Step 1: Fill the pitcher with water.

• Step 2: Add fruit pieces, such as strawberries, oranges, or cucumbers.

• Step 3: Refrigerate for several hours for a tasty and hydrating beverage.

Chapter Three

10 Special Occasion Menus For Celebrating Without Compromise On Health

1. Grilled Salmon with Quinoa Salad:

• Step 1: Marinate salmon fillets in olive oil, lemon juice, and herbs.

• Grill until done, then serve with a quinoa salad with veggies and herbs.

2. Roast Turkey and Steamed Vegetables:

• Step 1: Season a whole turkey with herbs and roast in the oven until golden brown.

• Step 2: Steam veggies such as broccoli, carrots, and green beans for a healthy side dish.

3. Vegetarian stir-fry with brown rice:

• Step 1: Cook tofu and veggies in a wok with garlic and ginger.

• Step 2: Serve with cooked brown rice for a fiber-rich and filling dinner.

4. Zucchini Noodles With Pesto And Grilled Chicken

• Begin by spiralizing zucchini into noodles and sautéing until soft.

• Step 2: Add homemade or store-bought pesto and grilled chicken strips for a low-carb pasta option.

5. Mushroom-Spinach Stuffed Chicken Breast:

• Step 1: Fill chicken breasts with sautéed mushrooms, spinach, and goat cheese.

• Step 2: Bake chicken until fully done, then serve with roasted veggies.

6. Cauliflower Crust Pizza:

• Step 1: Create a cauliflower crust by combining florets with egg and cheese.

• Step 2: Add marinara sauce, veggies, and lean protein, such as grilled chicken or turkey pepperoni.

- Step 3: Bake until the crust is crispy and the cheese is melted for guilt-free pizza.

7. Shrimp and Vegetable Skewer:

- Step 1: Thread shrimp and veggies on skewers, including bell peppers, onions, and zucchini.

- Step 2: Grill shrimp until pink and veggies are soft.

- Step 3: Pair with quinoa or brown rice for a complete dinner.

8. Lentil Soup with Whole Grain Bread:

- Step 1: Cook lentils, onions, carrots, and celery in vegetable broth until soft.

- Step 2: Season with herbs and spices (e.g. cumin, turmeric).

- Step 3: Pair with whole grain bread for a satisfying and healthy soup.

9. Stuffed bell peppers.

- Step 1: Cut bell peppers in half and remove seeds.

• Step 2: Add lean ground turkey or tofu, quinoa, and chopped veggies.

• Step 3: Bake until peppers are tender and the filling is fully cooked for a vibrant and tasty meal.

10. Salad Bar Buffet:

• Step 1: Create a buffet-style spread with various salad greens, toppings, and dressings.

• Step 2: Include protein-rich alternatives such as grilled chicken, hard-boiled eggs, beans, almonds, and seeds.

• Step 3: Allow visitors to personalize their salads to create a nutritious and fun dinner.

Healthy Eating Ideas For Newly Diagnosed Diabetics

• Plan nutritious meals with lean protein, healthy fats, fiber-rich carbs, and lots of veggies.

• Control portion sizes to prevent overeating and monitor carbohydrate consumption to maintain healthy blood sugar levels.

• Snack Smart: Eat nutrient-dense snacks like fruits, veggies, nuts, and yogurt to satiate hunger without creating blood sugar spikes.

• Stay Hydrated: Drink lots of water throughout the day for better digestion.

• Regular exercise may enhance insulin sensitivity and general health.

• Regularly monitor blood sugar levels and contact a healthcare practitioner to change food and medication accordingly.

• Seek Support: Consult a trained dietitian or join a diabetic support group to learn how to manage diabetes via food and lifestyle changes.

Understanding Carbs And Diabetes

• There are two sorts of carbohydrates: simple and complicated. Simple carbohydrates like sweets and processed grains may produce blood sugar increases, but complex carbs like whole grains, fruits, and vegetables digest more slowly.

• The glycemic index (GI) determines how rapidly meals elevate blood sugar levels. Choosing low-GI meals may assist in regulating blood sugar levels.

• Counting carbs in meals and snacks may help regulate blood sugar levels.

• Fiber-rich meals, such as whole grains, fruits, and vegetables, may help manage blood sugar levels by delaying digestion and increasing satiety.

• Balance carbs with protein, healthy fats, and fiber to reduce their influence on blood sugar levels.

Understanding Fats And Oils In Diabetic Diets

• Consume healthy fats like avocados, nuts, seeds, and olive oil in moderation to improve heart health and satiety.

• To lower the risk of heart disease, limit your consumption of saturated and trans fats from fatty meats, processed meals, and fried and packaged foods.

• To decrease inflammation and enhance lipid profiles, consume omega-3 fatty acids from fatty fish (e.g., salmon, mackerel, sardines) and flaxseeds.

• Choose healthier cooking oils, such as olive oil, avocado oil, and coconut oil, for improved heart health.

• Examine food labels for hidden fats and oils. Choose items with reduced saturated and trans fat levels.

10 Protein Options For Diabetic Meal Planning

1. Skinless Poultry: To reduce saturated fat consumption, use lean chicken or turkey parts that do not have skin.

2. Fatty fish such as salmon, mackerel, or trout include heart-healthy omega-3 fatty acids that may increase insulin sensitivity.

3. Lean Beef: To lower saturated fat intake, use "loin" or "round" cuts and remove visible fat.

4. Eggs: A flexible and inexpensive protein source, eggs include critical minerals such as vitamin D and choline.

5. Legumes: Beans, lentils, and chickpeas are plant-based protein sources high in fiber, which supports blood sugar regulation.

6. Tofu and tempeh are soy-based alternatives that offer a low-fat protein source for vegetarians and vegans.

7. Greek yogurt, which is high in protein and probiotics, is a pleasant snack or a foundation for sauces and dressings.

8. Cottage Cheese: Another dairy alternative, cottage cheese is low in carbs and strong in protein, making it a substantial meal or snack.

9. Nuts and Seeds: Almonds, walnuts, chia seeds, and flaxseeds provide protein and healthy fats, but portion management is essential owing to their high-calorie content.

10. Quinoa: A whole grain with a full amino acid profile, quinoa is a nutritional alternative to typical grains that may be included in diabetic meal plans.

10 Adding Fiber To Diabetic-Friendly Meals

1. veggies: Eat plenty of non-starchy veggies like spinach, broccoli, and bell peppers to boost fiber intake while keeping blood sugar stable.

2. Fruits: For more fiber, choose whole fruits over juices, focusing on berries, apples, and pears.

3. Whole Grains: Choose whole grains like oats, brown rice, and barley over processed grains since they include more fiber and vital minerals.

4. Legumes: Beans, lentils, and peas are high in protein and fiber, making them excellent complements to diabetic diets.

5. Nuts and Seeds: Add almonds, chia seeds, and flaxseeds to your meals or snacks for an added source of fiber and healthy fats.

6. Psyllium Husk: Including psyllium husk in dishes or drinks may greatly boost fiber content and improve digestive health.

7. Chia Seeds: When combined with liquid, chia seeds develop a gel-like consistency, providing fiber and texture to foods such as smoothies and puddings.

8. Avocados are high in fiber and contain healthful fats, making them a versatile element for salads, sandwiches, and toppings.

9. Popcorn: Air-popped popcorn is a low-calorie, high-fiber snack that may fulfill cravings without raising blood sugar levels.

10. Flaxseeds: Ground flaxseeds may be sprinkled over yogurt, porridge, or baked products to boost fiber content while retaining flavor.

Chapter Four

Balance Blood Sugar With Portion Control

Maintaining portion control is key for good blood sugar management. Here are a few tips:

• Use smaller plates to see portion quantities.

• Control carbohydrate intake by measuring starchy meals such as rice and pasta.

• Fill half of your plate with non-starchy veggies to increase bulk without adding calories.

• Limit calorie-dense condiments and sauces to prevent hidden sugars and fats.

• When eating out, limit portion sizes and share dishes or request a to-go box to store half for later.

• Aim for balanced snacks with protein, fiber, and healthy fats to maintain stable blood sugar levels between meals.

To properly regulate blood sugar levels, people with diabetes must pay close attention to their diets. While certain meals are good, others might hurt your diabetes. Here are 20 foods you should avoid to maintain stable blood sugar levels and general well-being:

1. Sugar-sweetened beverages include sodas, fruit juices, energy drinks, and sweetened tea. They are rich in sugar and may cause fast increases in blood glucose levels.

2. Candy & Sweets: Confections such as candy bars, chocolates, and sweet snacks contain refined sugars, which may rapidly raise blood sugar levels.

3. White bread and spaghetti are refined carbohydrates that the body rapidly breaks down into sugar, resulting in fast rises in blood glucose levels.

4. White rice, like white bread and pasta, is a refined carbohydrate that may induce high blood sugar levels.

5. Deep-fried meals, such as French fries and potato chips, contain significant quantities of harmful fats and carbs, which contribute to raised blood sugar levels.

6. Pastries & Baked Goods: Cakes, cookies, and pastries are often created with refined flour and sugars, making them unhealthy for diabetics.

7. High-Sugar Breakfast Cereals: Many breakfast cereals include sugar, which may cause significant spikes in blood glucose levels, particularly when ingested in high amounts.

8. Processed Meats: Processed meats, such as bacon, sausage, and deli meats, often have additional sugars and harmful fats, making them inappropriate for diabetes treatment.

9. Flavored Yogurts: Flavored yogurts may be rich in sugar and artificial ingredients, so stick with basic, unsweetened versions and add your flavorings.

10. Sweetened Condiments: Ketchup, barbecue sauce, and sweet chili sauce are common condiments that

contain hidden sugars; instead, go for low-sugar or sugar-free alternatives.

11. Canned Fruit in Syrup: While fruit is typically healthful, canned fruit in syrup has additional sugars, which may raise blood sugar levels. Choose fresh or canned fruit in water or natural juice instead.

12. Certain Fruits: Some fruits contain more sugar than others, which may cause abrupt rises in blood glucose levels. Grapes, mangos, and pineapple are among the examples.

13. Alcohol: Alcohol may disrupt blood sugar balance and produce hypoglycemia, particularly if drunk on an empty stomach or in significant quantities.

14. Full-Fat Dairy Products: While dairy may be part of a balanced diet, full-fat dairy products such as whole milk and cheese are rich in saturated fats, which may raise the risk of heart disease for diabetics.

15. High-Sodium Foods: Processed foods such as canned soups, salty snacks, and fast food meals are often high in

sodium, which may cause high blood pressure and raise the risk of heart disease.

16. Fried meals are often rich in harmful fats and may cause insulin resistance, making it difficult to control diabetes.

17. Sweetened Coffee beverages: Specialty coffee beverages such as frappuccinos and flavored lattes may include excessive quantities of sugar and harmful fats, resulting in blood glucose increases.

18. Certain morning foods, such as sweetened cereals, pancakes, and waffles, may produce rapid blood sugar increases owing to their high carbohydrate content.

19. Packaged Snack Foods: Snack foods such as crackers, pretzels, and granola bars often include refined carbs and added sugars, rendering them inappropriate for diabetic treatment.

20. Fast Food Meals: Fast food meals are often heavy in harmful fats, processed carbs, and salt, making them an unsuitable option for diabetics.

Individuals with diabetes may enhance their general health and well-being by avoiding these items and eating a diet rich in lean proteins, healthy fats, fiber, and complex carbs from whole grains, fruits, and vegetables. Remember to speak with a healthcare practitioner or registered dietitian for specialized dietary advice based on your unique circumstances and health objectives.

Meal Planning Strategies For Diabetics

1. Plan Ahead: Set aside time for meal planning and preparation to guarantee balanced meals throughout the week.

2. Focus on Whole Foods: To maintain stable blood sugar levels, base meals on lean meats, non-starchy veggies, whole grains, and healthy fats.

3. Spread Carbohydrates: To avoid blood sugar spikes, distribute carbohydrate consumption equally between meals and snacks.

4. Monitor Glycemic Index: Choose meals with a lower glycemic index to reduce blood glucose variations.

5. Experiment with Recipes: Look into diabetic-friendly options to make meals interesting and delectable while yet fulfilling nutritional requirements.

6. Portion Control: Use measuring cups, spoons, or visual aids to keep portion sizes under control and prevent overeating.

7. keep Hydrated: Drink lots of water throughout the day to keep hydrated and manage your appetite and blood sugar levels.

8. Listen to Your Body: Recognize hunger and fullness signals to avoid overeating and maintain a healthy weight.

9. Seek Help: For specialized meal planning advice and assistance, see a licensed dietitian or diabetes educator.

10. Maintain Consistency: Develop regular eating habits and meal times to ensure stable blood sugar management and general health.

Smart Shopping Tips For Diabetics

Grocery shopping is essential for diabetes management since it helps to maintain a balanced diet. Here are some recommendations to help diabetics make better decisions at the grocery store:

1. Plan Ahead: Before you go shopping, make a weekly food plan. This will allow you to create a list of precisely what you need, limiting the likelihood of impulsive purchases and ensuring you have the components for balanced meals.

2. Focus on entire Foods: Stock your basket with fruits, veggies, lean meats, and entire grains. These meals are high in nutrients and fiber, and low in added sugars, making them excellent options for blood sugar management.

3. Read the Labels: Always check the nutrition labels on packaged goods to see how much carbs, sugars, and fiber are included. To assist reduce blood glucose levels, look for goods that include less sugar and more fiber.

4. Choose foods with a low glycemic index (GI) to avoid blood sugar rises. Low GI diets include non-starchy vegetables, legumes, and whole grains such as quinoa and barley.

5. Limit Processed Foods: Processed foods often include hidden sugars, harmful fats, and excessive salt levels, which may impair blood sugar regulation and general health. Try to limit the quantity of processed foods you buy.

6. Stock up on Healthy Fats: Include avocados, almonds, seeds, and olive oil on your grocery list. These fats may increase insulin sensitivity and cardiovascular health.

7. Choose Lean Proteins: Lean protein sources include skinless chicken, fish, tofu, and lentils. These proteins have less saturated fats, which may help decrease the risk of heart disease, a major consequence of diabetes.

8. Portion proportions: When choosing meals, pay attention to portion proportions, particularly carbohydrate-rich items such as rice, pasta, and bread.

Portion control may help manage blood sugar and avoid overeating.

9. Shop the Perimeter: Fresh vegetables, lean proteins, and dairy goods are often found around the grocery store's perimeter. Shop around the perimeter to promote complete, nutrient-dense items.

10. Stay Hydrated: Remember to include beverages on your shopping list. Instead of sugary beverages such as soda or fruit juices, choose water, herbal teas, or sparkling water.

Chapter Five

Diabetes-Friendly Meal Planning

Meal planning may be a game changer for diabetics, allowing them to remain on track with their nutritional objectives while saving time and effort. Here's how to prepare meals effectively:

1. Choose dishes Wisely: Choose dishes that are balanced, healthy, and appropriate for your dietary requirements. Look for dishes that include a wide range of colorful veggies, lean meats, and healthy fats.

2. Prepare a Shopping List: Based on your selected recipes, make a detailed shopping list that contains all of the products you'll need for the week. This will improve your food shopping experience and eliminate last-minute trips to the market.

3. Set aside time each week for meal preparation. Set aside a few hours to prepare, divide up meals, and adequately store them for convenient access throughout the week.

4. Invest in Storage Containers: Purchase a selection of reusable storage containers of varying sizes to suit varied meal servings. Glass containers are great for reheating meals and are ecologically friendly.

5. Cook in bulk: Make big amounts of basic items such as cereals, proteins, and roasted veggies that can be combined to make various meals throughout the week. This saves time and ensures that you always have nutritious alternatives on hand.

6. measure Control: Use measuring cups, spoons, or a food scale to correctly measure out meals. This helps to limit calorie intake and reduces overeating, which may impact blood sugar levels.

7. Label and Date: Label each container with the dish's name and the date it was made. This makes it simple to recognize meals in the refrigerator or freezer and guarantees that you eat them before they spoil.

8. Include Snacks: Prepare nutritious snacks such as cut-up veggies, fruit slices, or portioned almonds to satisfy hunger between meals and avoid harmful snacking.

9. Rotate Your food: Keep mealtime interesting by changing your food every week. Experiment with varied dishes and tastes to avoid boredom and acquire a diversity of nutrients.

10. Stay Flexible: Make adjustments to your meal prep routine depending on your schedule, preferences, and any changes in your nutritional needs or health objectives.

10 Techniques For Healthier Diabetic Meals

1. Grilling is a healthy cooking technique that imparts flavor to meals without using excessive oils or fats. It is ideal for lean meats such as chicken, fish, and vegetables.

2. Steaming: Steaming maintains the natural tastes and nutrients of foods while using little additional fat. Vegetables, seafood, and grains such as rice and quinoa may all be cooked in a steamer basket or microwave.

3. Baking is a versatile cooking technique that allows you to make delicious, healthy meals with little added fat. Baking is useful for roasting vegetables, baking lean proteins, and even making whole-grain desserts.

4. Stir-frying is the process of quickly cooking ingredients in a small amount of oil over high heat. It's an excellent way to keep the crunchiness of vegetables while retaining their nutrients.

5. Broiling is similar to grilling, but it involves direct heat from above. It's a quick and easy way to cook proteins like fish or chicken breasts, giving them a flavorful crust with no added fats.

6. Poaching involves gently cooking foods in a simmering liquid, such as water or broth. It's a healthy way to prepare delicate proteins like fish or eggs without adding unnecessary calories.

7. Slow cooking allows flavors to develop over time with minimal hands-on effort. Use a slow cooker to make

hearty soups, stews, and tender cuts of meat with little added fat.

8. Sautéing is the process of quickly cooking ingredients in a small amount of oil over medium-high heat. It is ideal for cooking vegetables, lean meats, and tofu while retaining their natural flavors.

9. Griddling is the process of cooking foods on a flat surface with little or no added fat. It's ideal for caramelizing lean proteins like turkey burgers and vegetables.

10. Microwaving is a quick and easy cooking method that requires little added fat. Use the microwave to steam vegetables, cook grains, and reheat leftovers for a quick and healthy meal.

Chapter Six

What is Mindful Eating?

Mindful eating entails paying close attention to the sensory experience of eating, such as the taste, texture, and aroma of the food, as well as one's hunger and fullness indicators. It encourages nonjudgmental awareness of food choices and eating habits.

How Mindful Eating Can Help Manage Diabetes

1. Portion Control: Being mindful of portion sizes can help you avoid overeating and keep your blood sugar levels stable.

2. Food Choices: Mindful eating encourages the consumption of nutrient-dense foods that are beneficial to diabetes management, such as fruits, vegetables, lean proteins, and whole grains.

3. Eating Patterns: By being aware of their eating habits, people can avoid blood sugar spikes and dips throughout the day.

4. Emotional Eating: Mindful eating helps identify and address emotional eating triggers, lowering the risk of stress-induced overeating.

Practical Strategies For Mindful Eating

1. Slow Down: Take the time to chew your food thoroughly and savor each bite.

2. Eliminate Distractions: To focus on the eating experience, turn off television and electronic devices while eating.

3. Pay attention to hunger and fullness signals as you eat.

4. Practice Gratitude: Appreciate the flavors and nutrients provided by each meal.

Exercise's Role In Blood Sugar Management

Introduction: Regular exercise is an essential component of diabetes management because it improves insulin sensitivity and lowers blood sugar levels.

How Does Exercise Affect Blood Sugar?

1. Increased Insulin Sensitivity: Physical activity improves the body's ability to use insulin, resulting in better blood sugar control.

2. Exercise promotes the uptake of glucose by muscles for energy, which lowers blood sugar levels.

3. Weight Management: Regular exercise promotes a healthy weight, which is essential for diabetes management.

4. Stress Reduction: Exercise can reduce stress, which helps to regulate blood sugar levels.

Types Of Exercise For Diabetes

1. Aerobic exercise, such as walking, cycling, swimming, and dancing, benefits cardiovascular health and helps control blood sugar levels.

2. Strength Training: Weightlifting and other resistance exercises increase muscle mass, which aids in glucose uptake and metabolism.

3. Flexibility and Balance Exercises: Yoga and tai chi improve overall well-being and may indirectly help with blood sugar management.

Tips For Incorporating Exercise

1. Set Realistic Goals: Begin with achievable objectives and gradually increase the intensity and duration.

2. Maintain Consistency: Aim for regular exercise sessions of at least 150 minutes per week.

3. Monitor Blood Sugar Levels: Check your blood sugar before and after exercise to see how physical activity affects your glucose levels.

4. Stay Hydrated: Drink plenty of water before, during, and after exercising to avoid dehydration.

Stress Management Techniques for Diabetics

Introduction: Stress can have a significant impact on blood sugar levels, so stress management is essential for diabetes management.

1. Deep Breathing: Deep breathing exercises can help activate the body's relaxation response and lower stress hormones.

2. Mindfulness Meditation: Mindfulness meditation promotes present-moment awareness, which helps people cope with stress better.

3. Yoga and Tai Chi are mind-body practices that combine physical movement and breathing awareness to promote relaxation and stress reduction.

4. Progressive muscle relaxation is the process of tensing and relaxing muscle groups in sequence to release tension and promote relaxation.

5. Hobbies and Leisure Activities: To relax and recharge, do something you enjoy, such as reading, gardening, or listening to music.

1. Healthy Sleep Habits: Prioritize getting enough sleep, as lack of sleep can exacerbate stress and affect blood sugar levels.

2. Time Management: Good time management can help reduce feelings of overwhelm and stress, allowing for better diabetes self-care.

3. Social Support: Seek out friends, family, or support groups to share your experiences and get encouragement.

Sleep Hygiene and Its Effect on Blood Sugar

Introduction: Good sleep is essential for overall health and helps regulate blood sugar levels.

Chapter Seven

How Does Sleep Affect Blood Sugar

1. Insulin Sensitivity: Inadequate sleep can reduce insulin sensitivity, resulting in elevated blood sugar levels.

2. Hormonal Imbalance: Inadequate sleep disrupts hormone regulation, increasing stress hormones such as cortisol, which can raise blood sugar levels.

3. Sleep deprivation affects appetite-regulating hormones, which increases cravings for high-carbohydrate foods and may disrupt blood sugar control.

Tips To Improve Sleep Hygiene

1. Establish a Routine: Stick to a consistent sleep schedule by going to bed and waking up at the same time every day.

2. Create a Relaxing Environment: Make your bedroom conducive to sleep by reducing noise, light, and distractions.

3. Limit Screen Time: Avoid using electronic devices before bedtime because blue light exposure can disrupt sleep quality.

4. Avoid Stimulants: Limit your caffeine and alcohol consumption, especially in the hours before bedtime.

5. Relaxation Techniques: Before bed, unwind with activities such as reading, taking a warm bath, or doing gentle yoga.

Monitoring Blood Sugar Levels Effectively

Introduction: Regular blood sugar monitoring is essential for diabetes management because it provides valuable information about how lifestyle factors and medications influence glucose control.

Methods For Blood Sugar Monitoring

1. Self-Monitoring Blood Glucose (SMBG): Using a glucometer to check blood sugar levels at home, usually before and after meals and before bedtime.

2. Continuous Glucose Monitoring (CGM): CGM systems track blood sugar levels all day and night, providing real-time data and trends.

3. Hemoglobin A1c Test: This blood test measures average blood sugar levels over the previous 2-3 months, providing a complete picture of overall glucose control.

Nutritional Needs Of Diabetic Seniors

Dietary needs frequently change as people get older. Seniors with diabetes must pay close attention to their nutritional requirements. They may require fewer calories, but more nutrients, to maintain overall health. Adequate protein intake is critical for maintaining muscle mass and avoiding malnutrition. Furthermore, seniors with diabetes should eat whole grains, fruits, vegetables, lean proteins, and healthy fats to help control blood sugar levels and reduce the risk of complications.

Managing Diabetes And Coexisting Conditions With Diet

Many diabetics have additional health issues such as high blood pressure, high cholesterol, or heart disease. To manage these conditions in addition to diabetes, a well-balanced diet that promotes overall health is required.

A fiber-rich diet low in saturated fats and sodium, with plenty of fruits and vegetables, can help manage multiple health issues at once. Working closely with healthcare providers and dietitians to create a personalized meal plan is critical for successfully managing diabetes and coexisting conditions through diet.

Coping With Cravings And Temptations

Cravings and temptations can be difficult for diabetics to control, especially when trying to eat a healthy diet. Cravings can be managed through strategies such as mindful eating, keeping healthy snacks on hand, and finding healthier alternatives to favorite treats. Planning ahead of time and practicing portion control can also help you deal with cravings and stay on track with your diet.

Alcohol Consumption And The Effects On Blood Sugar

Individuals with diabetes should exercise caution when consuming alcohol because it has an impact on blood sugar levels. Drinking alcohol can cause blood sugar levels to rise or fall unexpectedly, depending on the type and amount of alcohol consumed, whether it is consumed with food, and personal factors such as medication use and overall health. Moderation is essential, and people should understand how alcohol affects their bodies and blood sugar levels.

Dining Tips For Social Gatherings And Events

Food is frequently the focal point of social gatherings and events, which can be difficult for diabetics. Planning, making wise choices from available options, and practicing portion control are all important strategies for navigating social situations while managing diabetes. Communicating your dietary requirements with hosts or restaurant staff can also help ensure that appropriate options are available.

Chapter Eight

Travel Tips For Diabetics

Traveling can disrupt regular meal schedules and access to familiar foods, making it difficult for diabetics to manage their condition. Planning ahead of time, packing necessary supplies, and researching food options at travel destinations can all help you keep your meal plan consistent while traveling. Additionally, diabetic travelers should stay hydrated, be aware of time zone changes, and bring snacks to avoid low blood sugar.

Meal Plan Changes For Weight Management

Maintaining a healthy weight is critical for managing diabetes and lowering the likelihood of complications. Portion control, nutrient-dense food selection, and calorie monitoring may all be necessary when adjusting meal plans to support weight management goals. Regular physical activity, in addition to dietary changes, can help with weight management.

Evaluating And Adapting Diabetes Meal Plans

Regularly evaluating and adapting diabetes meal plans is critical for meeting changing nutritional needs, controlling blood sugar levels, and achieving overall health objectives. Monitoring blood sugar levels, observing how different foods affect individual responses, and seeking advice from healthcare providers or dietitians can all help tailor meal plans to specific needs.

Conclusion

Understanding diabetics' specific dietary needs, managing coexisting conditions, dealing with challenges such as cravings and social situations, and making necessary meal plan adjustments are all part of providing nutritious meals. Diabetes patients can improve their overall health by focusing on balanced nutrition, mindful eating, and proactive management strategies.

Eating out presents unique challenges for diabetics due to a lack of control over portion sizes, ingredients, and cooking methods. Some dangers include:

1. Hidden Sugars and Carbohydrates: Restaurant meals frequently include hidden sugars and carbohydrates, which can cause blood sugar spikes. Sauces, dressings, and marinades may contain added sugars, whereas pasta and pizza are high in refined carbohydrates.

2. High salt Content: Many restaurant foods include a lot of salt, which may lead to high blood pressure and other health problems, particularly for diabetics who are more likely to develop heart disease.

3. Unhealthy Fats: Fried meals and dishes made with a lot of oil might be rich in unhealthy fats, which can harm your heart health and insulin sensitivity.

4. Limited Healthy selections: Some restaurants may offer few selections that are diabetic-friendly, making it difficult to make healthy choices.

5. Inconsistent Portion Sizes: Restaurant portion sizes are often greater than those suggested for diabetics, resulting in overeating and possible blood sugar increases.

To reduce these risks, people with diabetes should:

• Select eateries that provide healthier alternatives or customized menu items.

• Request dish adjustments, such as switching vegetables for starches or ordering dressings and sauces separately.

• Minimize portion sizes and share meals or pack leftovers.

• Monitor blood sugar levels before and after dining out to see how restaurant meals affect blood sugar management.

• Review meals online and make educated selections based on dietary preferences and nutritional requirements.